Week:_____ From: To:

Weekly Plan

	MAEL	Activity	Calories Burned	Note
Sunday				
Monday				
Tuesday				
Wednesday				
Thursday				
Friday				
Saturday				

Today's Plan

Activity to Do:

Food Journal

	Food /Beverage	calories
1		
2		
3		
4		
5		
6		
7		
8		
9		
10		
11		
12		

Total:

Total Activity:_________ Min. **Burned:**_________ Kcal

Water Intake

DATE: / /

Today's Plan

Food Journal

	Food /Beverage	calories
1		
2		
3		
4		
5		
6		
7		
8		
9		
10		
11		
12		

Total:

Total Activity: __________ Min.   Burned: __________ Kcal

Water Intake

Today's Plan

Activity to Do:

Food Journal

	Food /Beverage	calories
1		
2		
3		
4		
5		
6		
7		
8		
9		
10		
11		
12		

Total:

Total Activity: _______ Min.   Burned: ___________ Kcal

Water Intake

DATE: /   /

Today's Plan

Activity to Do:

Food Journal

	Food /Beverage	calories
1		
2		
3		
4		
5		
6		
7		
8		
9		
10		
11		
12		

Total:	

Total Activity: _________ Min.   Burned: _________ Kcal

Water Intake

Today's Plan

Activity to Do:

Food Journal

	Food /Beverage	calories
1		
2		
3		
4		
5		
6		
7		
8		
9		
10		
11		
12		

Total:

Total Activity: _________ Min.   Burned: _____________ Kcal

Water Intake

DATE: /   /

Today's Plan

Activity to Do:

Food Journal

	Food /Beverage	calories
1		
2		
3		
4		
5		
6		
7		
8		
9		
10		
11		
12		

Total:	

Total Activity:_________ Min. Burned:____________ Kcal

Water Intake

DATE: /   /

Today's Plan

Food Journal

	Food /Beverage	calories
1		
2		
3		
4		
5		
6		
7		
8		
9		
10		
11		
12		

Total:

Total Activity: __________ Min.   Burned: __________ Kcal

Water Intake

Week:____ From: To:

Weekly Summary

	MAEL	Activity	Calories Burned	Note
Sunday	☺ ☹	☺ ☹	☺ ☹	
Monday	☺ ☹	☺ ☹	☺ ☹	
Tuesday	☺ ☹	☺ ☹	☺ ☹	
Wednesday	☺ ☹	☺ ☹	☺ ☹	
Thursday	☺ ☹	☺ ☹	☺ ☹	
Friday	☺ ☹	☺ ☹	☺ ☹	
Saturday	☺ ☹	☺ ☹	☺ ☹	

Note

Week:____ From: To:

Weekly Plan

	MAEL	Activity	Calories Burned	Note
Sunday				
Monday				
Tuesday				
Wednesday				
Thursday				
Friday				
Saturday				

Today's Plan

Activity to Do:

Food Journal

	Food /Beverage	calories
1		
2		
3		
4		
5		
6		
7		
8		
9		
10		
11		
12		

Total:	

Total Activity:_________ Min. Burned:_____________ Kcal

Water Intake

Today's Plan

<table>
<tr><td rowspan="9">Activity to Do:</td><td>○ ....</td></tr>
<tr><td>○ ....</td></tr>
<tr><td>○ ....</td></tr>
<tr><td>○ ....</td></tr>
<tr><td>○ ....</td></tr>
<tr><td>○ ....</td></tr>
<tr><td>○ ....</td></tr>
<tr><td>○ ....</td></tr>
<tr><td>○ ....</td></tr>
</table>

Food Journal

	Food /Beverage	calories
1		
2		
3		
4		
5		
6		
7		
8		
9		
10		
11		
12		

	Total:	

Total Activity:_________ Min. | Burned:____________ Kcal

Water Intake ▽ ▽ ▽ ▽ ▽ ▽ ▽ ▽

Today's Plan

<table>
<tr><td rowspan="9" style="writing-mode: vertical-lr">Activity to Do:</td></tr>
</table>

○ ....
○ ....
○ ....
○ ....
○ ....
○ ....
○ ....
○ ....
○ ....

Food Journal

	Food /Beverage	calories
1		
2		
3		
4		
5		
6		
7		
8		
9		
10		
11		
12		

Total:	

Total Activity: _________ Min. | Burned: _____________ Kcal

Water Intake ▭ ▭ ▭ ▭ ▭ ▭ ▭ ▭

DATE: / /

Today's Plan

Food Journal

	Food /Beverage	calories
1		
2		
3		
4		
5		
6		
7		
8		
9		
10		
11		
12		

Total:	

Total Activity:_________ Min.   Burned:___________ Kcal

Water Intake

DATE: / /

Today's Plan

Activity to Do:

Food Journal

	Food /Beverage	calories
1		
2		
3		
4		
5		
6		
7		
8		
9		
10		
11		
12		

Total:

Total Activity:__________ Min.   Burned:__________ Kcal

Water Intake

DATE: /   /

Today's Plan

Food Journal

	Food /Beverage	calories
1		
2		
3		
4		
5		
6		
7		
8		
9		
10		
11		
12		

Total:	

Total Activity: _________ Min.   Burned: _________ Kcal

Water Intake

Today's Plan

Activity to Do:

Food Journal

#	Food /Beverage	calories
1		
2		
3		
4		
5		
6		
7		
8		
9		
10		
11		
12		

Total:	

Total Activity: _________ Min.   Burned: _________ Kcal

Water Intake

Week:_____ From: To:

Weekly Summary

	MAEL	Activity	Calories Burned	Note
Sunday	☺ ☹	☺ ☹	☺ ☹	
Monday	☺ ☹	☺ ☹	☺ ☹	
Tuesday	☺ ☹	☺ ☹	☺ ☹	
Wednesday	☺ ☹	☺ ☹	☺ ☹	
Thursday	☺ ☹	☺ ☹	☺ ☹	
Friday	☺ ☹	☺ ☹	☺ ☹	
Saturday	☺ ☹	☺ ☹	☺ ☹	

Note

Week:____ From: To:

Weekly Plan

	MAEL	Activity	Calories Burned	Note
Sunday				
Monday				
Tuesday				
Wednesday				
Thursday				
Friday				
Saturday				

Today's Plan

Activity to Do:

Food Journal

	Food /Beverage	calories
1		
2		
3		
4		
5		
6		
7		
8		
9		
10		
11		
12		

Total:	

Total Activity:___________ Min.   Burned:___________ Kcal

Water Intake

DATE: / /

Today's Plan

Food Journal

	Food /Beverage	calories
1		
2		
3		
4		
5		
6		
7		
8		
9		
10		
11		
12		

Total:	

Total Activity:________ Min.   Burned:__________ Kcal

Water Intake

DATE: /   /

Today's Plan

Food Journal

	Food /Beverage	calories
1		
2		
3		
4		
5		
6		
7		
8		
9		
10		
11		
12		

Total:

Total Activity: __________ Min.   Burned: __________ Kcal

Water Intake

DATE: /   /

Today's Plan

Activity to Do:

Food Journal

	Food /Beverage	calories
1		
2		
3		
4		
5		
6		
7		
8		
9		
10		
11		
12		

Total:

Total Activity: _______ Min.   Burned: _________ Kcal

Water Intake

DATE: /   /

Today's Plan

Activity to Do:

Food Journal

	Food /Beverage	calories
1		
2		
3		
4		
5		
6		
7		
8		
9		
10		
11		
12		

Total:	

Total Activity: _________ Min.   Burned: _________ Kcal

Water Intake

DATE: / /

Today's Plan

Activity to Do:

Food Journal

	Food /Beverage	calories
1		
2		
3		
4		
5		
6		
7		
8		
9		
10		
11		
12		

Total:

Total Activity: _________ Min.   Burned: _________ Kcal

Water Intake

Today's Plan

Activity to Do:

Food Journal

	Food /Beverage	calories
1		
2		
3		
4		
5		
6		
7		
8		
9		
10		
11		
12		

Total:	

Total Activity:__________ Min.   Burned:______________ Kcal

Water Intake

Week:____ From: To:

Weekly Summary

	MAEL	Activity	Calories Burned	Note
Sunday	🙂 ☹️	🙂 ☹️	🙂 ☹️	
Monday	🙂 ☹️	🙂 ☹️	🙂 ☹️	
Tuesday	🙂 ☹️	🙂 ☹️	🙂 ☹️	
Wednesday	🙂 ☹️	🙂 ☹️	🙂 ☹️	
Thursday	🙂 ☹️	🙂 ☹️	🙂 ☹️	
Friday	🙂 ☹️	🙂 ☹️	🙂 ☹️	
Saturday	🙂 ☹️	🙂 ☹️	🙂 ☹️	

Note

Week:_____ From: To:

Weekly Plan

	MAEL	Activity	Calories Burned	Note
Sunday				
Monday				
Tuesday				
Wednesday				
Thursday				
Friday				
Saturday				

DATE: /   /

Today's Plan

Food Journal

	Food /Beverage	calories
1		
2		
3		
4		
5		
6		
7		
8		
9		
10		
11		
12		

Total:	

Total Activity: _________ Min.   Burned: _________ Kcal

Water Intake

DATE: / /

Today's Plan

Activity to Do:

○ ....
○ ....
○ ....
○ ....
○ ....
○ ....
○ ....
○ ....
○ ....

Food Journal

	Food /Beverage	calories
1		
2		
3		
4		
5		
6		
7		
8		
9		
10		
11		
12		

Total:	

Total Activity: _________ Min.   Burned: ___________ Kcal

Water Intake ▢ ▢ ▢ ▢ ▢ ▢ ▢ ▢

Today's Plan

Activity to Do:

Food Journal

	Food /Beverage	calories
1		
2		
3		
4		
5		
6		
7		
8		
9		
10		
11		
12		

Total:

Total Activity: _______ Min. Burned: _______ Kcal

Water Intake

DATE: / /

Today's Plan

Food Journal

	Food /Beverage	calories
1		
2		
3		
4		
5		
6		
7		
8		
9		
10		
11		
12		

Total:	

Total Activity: _________ Min. Burned: _________ Kcal

Water Intake

DATE: /   /

Today's Plan

Activity to Do:

Food Journal

	Food /Beverage	calories
1		
2		
3		
4		
5		
6		
7		
8		
9		
10		
11		
12		

Total:

Total Activity: _________ **Min.**   **Burned:** _____________ **Kcal**

Water Intake

DATE: /   /

Today's Plan

Activity to Do:

Food Journal

	Food /Beverage	calories
1		
2		
3		
4		
5		
6		
7		
8		
9		
10		
11		
12		

Total:

Total Activity: _________ Min.   Burned: _________ Kcal

Water Intake

Today's Plan

Activity to Do:

Food Journal

	Food /Beverage	calories
1		
2		
3		
4		
5		
6		
7		
8		
9		
10		
11		
12		

Total:

Total Activity: _________ **Min.** **Burned:** _________ **Kcal**

Water Intake

Week:____ From: To:

Weekly Summary

	MAEL	Activity	Calories Burned	Note
Sunday				
Monday				
Tuesday				
Wednesday				
Thursday				
Friday				
Saturday				

Note

Week:____ From: To:

Weekly Plan

	MAEL	Activity	Calories Burned	Note
Sunday				
Monday				
Tuesday				
Wednesday				
Thursday				
Friday				
Saturday				

Today's Plan

Activity to Do:

Food Journal

	Food /Beverage	calories
1		
2		
3		
4		
5		
6		
7		
8		
9		
10		
11		
12		

Total:	

Total Activity: _________ Min.   Burned: _________ Kcal

Water Intake

DATE: /   /

Today's Plan

Food Journal

	Food /Beverage	calories
1		
2		
3		
4		
5		
6		
7		
8		
9		
10		
11		
12		

Total:

Total Activity:_________ Min.   Burned:_____________ Kcal

Water Intake

Today's Plan

Activity to Do:

Food Journal

	Food /Beverage	calories
1		
2		
3		
4		
5		
6		
7		
8		
9		
10		
11		
12		

Total:

Total Activity: _______ Min.   **Burned:** _______ Kcal

Water Intake

DATE: /   /

Today's Plan

Activity to Do:

Food Journal

	Food /Beverage	calories
1		
2		
3		
4		
5		
6		
7		
8		
9		
10		
11		
12		

Total:

Total Activity:_________ Min.   Burned:___________ Kcal

Water Intake

Today's Plan

Activity to Do:

Food Journal

	Food /Beverage	calories
1		
2		
3		
4		
5		
6		
7		
8		
9		
10		
11		
12		

Total:	

Total Activity: __________ Min. Burned: __________ Kcal

Water Intake

DATE: /   /

Today's Plan

Activity to Do:

Food Journal

	Food /Beverage	calories
1		
2		
3		
4		
5		
6		
7		
8		
9		
10		
11		
12		

Total:	

Total Activity: _________ Min.   Burned: _________ Kcal

Water Intake

Today's Plan

Activity to Do:

Food Journal

	Food /Beverage	calories
1		
2		
3		
4		
5		
6		
7		
8		
9		
10		
11		
12		

Total:

Total Activity: __________ Min.   Burned: __________ Kcal

Water Intake

Week:_____ From: To:

Weekly Summary

	MAEL	Activity	Calories Burned	Note
Sunday	🙂 ☹️	🙂 ☹️	🙂 ☹️	
Monday	🙂 ☹️	🙂 ☹️	🙂 ☹️	
Tuesday	🙂 ☹️	🙂 ☹️	🙂 ☹️	
Wednesday	🙂 ☹️	🙂 ☹️	🙂 ☹️	
Thursday	🙂 ☹️	🙂 ☹️	🙂 ☹️	
Friday	🙂 ☹️	🙂 ☹️	🙂 ☹️	
Saturday	🙂 ☹️	🙂 ☹️	🙂 ☹️	

Note

Week:____ From: To:

Weekly Plan

	MAEL	Activity	Calories Burned	Note
Sunday				
Monday				
Tuesday				
Wednesday				
Thursday				
Friday				
Saturday				

DATE: /   /

Today's Plan

Food Journal

	Food /Beverage	calories
1		
2		
3		
4		
5		
6		
7		
8		
9		
10		
11		
12		

Total:	

Total Activity: _________ Min.   Burned: _____________ Kcal

Water Intake

DATE: / /

Today's Plan

Activity to Do:

○ ....
○ ....
○ ....
○ ....
○ ....
○ ....
○ ....
○ ....
○ ....
○ ....

Food Journal

	Food /Beverage	calories
1		
2		
3		
4		
5		
6		
7		
8		
9		
10		
11		
12		

Total:

Total Activity: _________ Min.   Burned: ___________ Kcal

Water Intake

DATE: / /

Today's Plan

Food Journal

	Food /Beverage	calories
1		
2		
3		
4		
5		
6		
7		
8		
9		
10		
11		
12		

Total:

Total Activity:________ Min.   Burned:____________ Kcal

Water Intake

DATE: /   /

Today's Plan

Food Journal

	Food /Beverage	calories
1		
2		
3		
4		
5		
6		
7		
8		
9		
10		
11		
12		

Total:

Total Activity: _________ Min.   Burned: __________ Kcal

Water Intake

DATE: / /

Today's Plan

Food Journal

	Food /Beverage	calories
1		
2		
3		
4		
5		
6		
7		
8		
9		
10		
11		
12		

Total:	

Total Activity:___________ Min.   Burned:____________ Kcal

Water Intake

DATE: /   /

Today's Plan

Activity to Do:

Food Journal

	Food /Beverage	calories
1		
2		
3		
4		
5		
6		
7		
8		
9		
10		
11		
12		

Total:

Total Activity:________ Min.   Burned:__________ Kcal

Water Intake

DATE: / /

Today's Plan

Activity to Do:

○
○
○
○
○
○
○
○
○

Food Journal

	Food /Beverage	calories
1		
2		
3		
4		
5		
6		
7		
8		
9		
10		
11		
12		

Total:	

Total Activity:__________ Min. Burned:__________ Kcal

Water Intake

Week:_____ From: To:

Weekly Summary

	MAEL	Activity	Calories Burned	Note
Sunday	☺ ☹	☺ ☹	☺ ☹	
Monday	☺ ☹	☺ ☹	☺ ☹	
Tuesday	☺ ☹	☺ ☹	☺ ☹	
Wednesday	☺ ☹	☺ ☹	☺ ☹	
Thursday	☺ ☹	☺ ☹	☺ ☹	
Friday	☺ ☹	☺ ☹	☺ ☹	
Saturday	☺ ☹	☺ ☹	☺ ☹	

Note

Week:____ From: To:

Weekly Plan

	MAEL	Activity	Calories Burned	Note
Sunday				
Monday				
Tuesday				
Wednesday				
Thursday				
Friday				
Saturday				

DATE: / /

Today's Plan

Activity to Do:

Food Journal

	Food /Beverage	calories
1		
2		
3		
4		
5		
6		
7		
8		
9		
10		
11		
12		

Total:	

Total Activity: _________ Min. | Burned: _________ Kcal

Water Intake

DATE: /   /

Today's Plan

Food Journal

	Food /Beverage	calories
1		
2		
3		
4		
5		
6		
7		
8		
9		
10		
11		
12		

Total:	

Total Activity: _________ Min.   Burned: _____________ Kcal

Water Intake

DATE: / /

Today's Plan

Activity to Do:

Food Journal

	Food /Beverage	calories
1		
2		
3		
4		
5		
6		
7		
8		
9		
10		
11		
12		

Total:	

Total Activity:_________ Min.   Burned:_________ Kcal

Water Intake

Today's Plan

Food Journal

	Food /Beverage	calories
1		
2		
3		
4		
5		
6		
7		
8		
9		
10		
11		
12		

Total:	

Total Activity: __________ Min. | Burned: __________ Kcal

Water Intake

DATE: /   /

Today's Plan

Activity to Do:

Food Journal

	Food /Beverage	calories
1		
2		
3		
4		
5		
6		
7		
8		
9		
10		
11		
12		

Total:	

Total Activity: __________ Min.   Burned: __________ Kcal

Water Intake

Today's Plan

Activity to Do:

○
○
○
○
○
○
○
○
○

Food Journal

	Food /Beverage	calories
1		
2		
3		
4		
5		
6		
7		
8		
9		
10		
11		
12		

Total:	

Total Activity: _________ Min.   Burned: _____________ Kcal

Water Intake

DATE: / /

Today's Plan

Food Journal

	Food /Beverage	calories
1		
2		
3		
4		
5		
6		
7		
8		
9		
10		
11		
12		

Total:

Total Activity:_________ Min. Burned:_________ Kcal

Water Intake

Week:______ From: To:

Weekly Summary

	MAEL	Activity	Calories Burned	Note
Sunday	☺ ☹	☺ ☹	☺ ☹	
Monday	☺ ☹	☺ ☹	☺ ☹	
Tuesday	☺ ☹	☺ ☹	☺ ☹	
Wednesday	☺ ☹	☺ ☹	☺ ☹	
Thursday	☺ ☹	☺ ☹	☺ ☹	
Friday	☺ ☹	☺ ☹	☺ ☹	
Saturday	☺ ☹	☺ ☹	☺ ☹	

Note

Week:____ From: To:

Weekly Plan

	MAEL	Activity	Calories Burned	Note
Sunday				
Monday				
Tuesday				
Wednesday				
Thursday				
Friday				
Saturday				

DATE: /   /

Today's Plan

Food Journal

	Food /Beverage	calories
1		
2		
3		
4		
5		
6		
7		
8		
9		
10		
11		
12		

Total:	

Total Activity: _________ Min.   Burned: _____________ Kcal

Water Intake

DATE: /   /

Today's Plan

Activity to Do:

- ○
- ○
- ○
- ○
- ○
- ○
- ○
- ○
- ○
- ○

Food Journal

	Food /Beverage	calories
1		
2		
3		
4		
5		
6		
7		
8		
9		
10		
11		
12		

Total:

Total Activity: _______ Min.   Burned: _________ Kcal

Water Intake

Today's Plan

Activity to Do:

Food Journal

	Food /Beverage	calories
1		
2		
3		
4		
5		
6		
7		
8		
9		
10		
11		
12		

Total:

Total Activity: __________ Min. Burned: __________ Kcal

Water Intake

DATE: /   /

Today's Plan

Activity to Do:

○ ....
○ ....
○ ....
○ ....
○ ....
○ ....
○ ....
○ ....

Food Journal

	Food /Beverage	calories
1		
2		
3		
4		
5		
6		
7		
8		
9		
10		
11		
12		

Total:	

Total Activity: _________ Min.   Burned: _________ Kcal

Water Intake ▢ ▢ ▢ ▢ ▢ ▢ ▢ ▢

DATE: / /

Today's Plan

Activity to Do:

Food Journal

	Food /Beverage	calories
1		
2		
3		
4		
5		
6		
7		
8		
9		
10		
11		
12		

Total:	

Total Activity:_________ Min.   Burned:_____________ Kcal

Water Intake

DATE: / /

Today's Plan

Activity to Do:

○ ....
○ ....
○ ....
○ ....
○ ....
○ ....
○ ....
○ ....
○ ....

Food Journal

	Food /Beverage	calories
1		
2		
3		
4		
5		
6		
7		
8		
9		
10		
11		
12		

Total:	

Total Activity:_________ Min.   Burned:_________ Kcal

Water Intake ⬜ ⬜ ⬜ ⬜ ⬜ ⬜ ⬜ ⬜

DATE: /   /

Today's Plan

Activity to Do:

Food Journal

	Food /Beverage	calories
1		
2		
3		
4		
5		
6		
7		
8		
9		
10		
11		
12		

Total:	

Total Activity:___________ Min.   Burned:_____________ Kcal

Water Intake

Week:____ From: To:

Weekly Summary

	MAEL	Activity	Calories Burned	Note
Sunday	🙂 ☹️	🙂 ☹️	🙂 ☹️	
Monday	🙂 ☹️	🙂 ☹️	🙂 ☹️	
Tuesday	🙂 ☹️	🙂 ☹️	🙂 ☹️	
Wednesday	🙂 ☹️	🙂 ☹️	🙂 ☹️	
Thursday	🙂 ☹️	🙂 ☹️	🙂 ☹️	
Friday	🙂 ☹️	🙂 ☹️	🙂 ☹️	
Saturday	🙂 ☹️	🙂 ☹️	🙂 ☹️	

Note

Week:____ From: To:

Weekly Plan

	MAEL	Activity	Calories Burned	Note
Sunday				
Monday				
Tuesday				
Wednesday				
Thursday				
Friday				
Saturday				

DATE: / /

Today's Plan

Activity to Do:

Food Journal

	Food /Beverage	calories
1		
2		
3		
4		
5		
6		
7		
8		
9		
10		
11		
12		

Total:	

Total Activity:_________ Min. Burned:___________ Kcal

Water Intake

DATE: /   /

Today's Plan

Activity to Do:

○
○
○
○
○
○
○
○
○
○

Food Journal

	Food /Beverage	calories
1		
2		
3		
4		
5		
6		
7		
8		
9		
10		
11		
12		

Total:	

Total Activity: _________ Min.   Burned: _________ Kcal

Water Intake

DATE: /   /

Today's Plan

Activity to Do:

Food Journal

	Food /Beverage	calories
1		
2		
3		
4		
5		
6		
7		
8		
9		
10		
11		
12		

Total:	

Total Activity:_________ Min. Burned:_____________ Kcal

Water Intake

DATE: / /

Today's Plan

Food Journal

	Food /Beverage	calories
1		
2		
3		
4		
5		
6		
7		
8		
9		
10		
11		
12		

Total:	

Total Activity:_________ Min.   Burned:______________ Kcal

Water Intake

Today's Plan

Activity to Do:

Food Journal

	Food /Beverage	calories
1		
2		
3		
4		
5		
6		
7		
8		
9		
10		
11		
12		

Total:	

Total Activity:________ Min.   Burned:__________ Kcal

Water Intake

DATE: /   /

Today's Plan

Activity to Do:

Food Journal

	Food /Beverage	calories
1		
2		
3		
4		
5		
6		
7		
8		
9		
10		
11		
12		

Total:	

Total Activity: _________ Min.   Burned: _____________ Kcal

Water Intake

Today's Plan

Activity to Do:

Food Journal

	Food /Beverage	calories
1		
2		
3		
4		
5		
6		
7		
8		
9		
10		
11		
12		

Total:	

Total Activity:_________ Min.   Burned:_____________ Kcal

Water Intake

Week:_____ From: To:

Weekly Summary

	MAEL	Activity	Calories Burned	Note
Sunday	😊 ☹️	😊 ☹️	😊 ☹️	
Monday	😊 ☹️	😊 ☹️	😊 ☹️	
Tuesday	😊 ☹️	😊 ☹️	😊 ☹️	
Wednesday	😊 ☹️	😊 ☹️	😊 ☹️	
Thursday	😊 ☹️	😊 ☹️	😊 ☹️	
Friday	😊 ☹️	😊 ☹️	😊 ☹️	
Saturday	😊 ☹️	😊 ☹️	😊 ☹️	

Note

Week:____ From: To:

Weekly Plan

	MAEL	Activity	Calories Burned	Note
Sunday				
Monday				
Tuesday				
Wednesday				
Thursday				
Friday				
Saturday				

DATE: / /

Today's Plan

Food Journal

	Food /Beverage	calories
1		
2		
3		
4		
5		
6		
7		
8		
9		
10		
11		
12		

Total:

Total Activity: _________ Min.   Burned: _____________ Kcal

Water Intake

DATE: /   /

Today's Plan

Activity to Do:

- ○ ....
- ○ ....
- ○ ....
- ○ ....
- ○ ....
- ○ ....
- ○ ....
- ○ ....
- ○ ....

Food Journal

	Food /Beverage	calories
1		
2		
3		
4		
5		
6		
7		
8		
9		
10		
11		
12		

Total:

Total Activity:_________ Min.   Burned:___________ Kcal

Water Intake

DATE: /   /

Today's Plan

Food Journal

	Food /Beverage	calories
1		
2		
3		
4		
5		
6		
7		
8		
9		
10		
11		
12		

Total:	

Total Activity: _________ Min. | Burned: _____________ Kcal

Water Intake

DATE: / /

Today's Plan

Food Journal

	Food /Beverage	calories
1		
2		
3		
4		
5		
6		
7		
8		
9		
10		
11		
12		

Total:	

Total Activity: _________ Min.   Burned: _________ Kcal

Water Intake

DATE: /   /

Today's Plan

Activity to Do:

Food Journal

	Food /Beverage	calories
1		
2		
3		
4		
5		
6		
7		
8		
9		
10		
11		
12		

Total:	

Total Activity: _________ Min.   Burned: _____________ Kcal

Water Intake

DATE: /   /

Today's Plan

Food Journal

	Food /Beverage	calories
1		
2		
3		
4		
5		
6		
7		
8		
9		
10		
11		
12		

Total:	

Total Activity: ________ Min.   Burned: ________ Kcal

Water Intake

DATE: / /

Today's Plan

Activity to Do:

○
○
○
○
○
○
○
○
○
○

Food Journal

	Food /Beverage	calories
1		
2		
3		
4		
5		
6		
7		
8		
9		
10		
11		
12		

Total:

Total Activity: _______ Min.   Burned: _______ Kcal

Water Intake

Week:____ From: To:

Weekly Summary

	MAEL	Activity	Calories Burned	Note
Sunday	☺ ☹	☺ ☹	☺ ☹	
Monday	☺ ☹	☺ ☹	☺ ☹	
Tuesday	☺ ☹	☺ ☹	☺ ☹	
Wednesday	☺ ☹	☺ ☹	☺ ☹	
Thursday	☺ ☹	☺ ☹	☺ ☹	
Friday	☺ ☹	☺ ☹	☺ ☹	
Saturday	☺ ☹	☺ ☹	☺ ☹	

Note

Week:____ From: To:

Weekly Plan

	MAEL	Activity	Calories Burned	Note
Sunday				
Monday				
Tuesday				
Wednesday				
Thursday				
Friday				
Saturday				

DATE: /   /

Today's Plan

Activity to Do:

Food Journal

#	Food /Beverage	calories
1		
2		
3		
4		
5		
6		
7		
8		
9		
10		
11		
12		

Total:	

Total Activity:_________ Min. Burned: _____________ Kcal

Water Intake

DATE: /   /

Today's Plan

Activity to Do:

Food Journal

	Food /Beverage	calories
1		
2		
3		
4		
5		
6		
7		
8		
9		
10		
11		
12		

Total:	

Total Activity:_________ Min.   Burned:_________ Kcal

Water Intake

DATE: / /

Today's Plan

Activity to Do:

Food Journal

	Food /Beverage	calories
1		
2		
3		
4		
5		
6		
7		
8		
9		
10		
11		
12		

Total:	

Total Activity: __________ Min. Burned: __________ Kcal

Water Intake

Today's Plan

Activity to Do:

Food Journal

	Food /Beverage	calories
1		
2		
3		
4		
5		
6		
7		
8		
9		
10		
11		
12		

Total:	

Total Activity: _________ Min. Burned: ___________ Kcal

Water Intake

Today's Plan

Activity to Do:

○
○
○
○
○
○
○
○
○

Food Journal

	Food /Beverage	calories
1		
2		
3		
4		
5		
6		
7		
8		
9		
10		
11		
12		

Total:	

Total Activity: _________ Min. Burned: _____________ Kcal

Water Intake

DATE: / /

Today's Plan

Activity to Do:

- ○
- ○
- ○
- ○
- ○
- ○
- ○
- ○
- ○

Food Journal

	Food /Beverage	calories
1		
2		
3		
4		
5		
6		
7		
8		
9		
10		
11		
12		

Total:	

Total Activity: ________ Min. | Burned: ____________ Kcal

Water Intake ☐ ☐ ☐ ☐ ☐ ☐ ☐ ☐

DATE: / /

Today's Plan

Food Journal

	Food /Beverage	calories
1		
2		
3		
4		
5		
6		
7		
8		
9		
10		
11		
12		

Total:

Total Activity: ______ Min.   Burned: ______ Kcal

Water Intake

Week:_____ From: To:

Weekly Summary

	MAEL	Activity	Calories Burned	Note
Sunday	☺ ☹	☺ ☹	☺ ☹	
Monday	☺ ☹	☺ ☹	☺ ☹	
Tuesday	☺ ☹	☺ ☹	☺ ☹	
Wednesday	☺ ☹	☺ ☹	☺ ☹	
Thursday	☺ ☹	☺ ☹	☺ ☹	
Friday	☺ ☹	☺ ☹	☺ ☹	
Saturday	☺ ☹	☺ ☹	☺ ☹	

Note

Week:___ From: To:

Weekly Plan

	MAEL	Activity	Calories Burned	Note
Sunday				
Monday				
Tuesday				
Wednesday				
Thursday				
Friday				
Saturday				

DATE: /   /

Today's Plan

Activity to Do:

Food Journal

	Food /Beverage	calories
1		
2		
3		
4		
5		
6		
7		
8		
9		
10		
11		
12		

Total:	

Total Activity:__________ Min.   Burned:____________ Kcal

Water Intake

DATE: /   /

Today's Plan

Activity to Do:

Food Journal

	Food /Beverage	calories
1		
2		
3		
4		
5		
6		
7		
8		
9		
10		
11		
12		

Total:	

Total Activity: _________ Min.   Burned: _________ Kcal

Water Intake

DATE: / /

Today's Plan

Activity to Do:

Food Journal

	Food /Beverage	calories
1		
2		
3		
4		
5		
6		
7		
8		
9		
10		
11		
12		

Total:	

Total Activity: __________ Min.   Burned: __________ Kcal

Water Intake

DATE: / /

Today's Plan

Activity to Do:

Food Journal

	Food /Beverage	calories
1		
2		
3		
4		
5		
6		
7		
8		
9		
10		
11		
12		

Total:	

Total Activity: _________ Min. Burned: __________ Kcal

Water Intake

DATE: / /

Today's Plan

Activity to Do:

Food Journal

	Food /Beverage	calories
1		
2		
3		
4		
5		
6		
7		
8		
9		
10		
11		
12		

Total:

Total Activity: _______ Min.   Burned: _______ Kcal

Water Intake

DATE: / /

Today's Plan

Activity to Do:

Food Journal

	Food /Beverage	calories
1		
2		
3		
4		
5		
6		
7		
8		
9		
10		
11		
12		

Total:

Total Activity:_________ Min. Burned:____________ Kcal

Water Intake

DATE: / /

Today's Plan

Food Journal

	Food /Beverage	calories
1		
2		
3		
4		
5		
6		
7		
8		
9		
10		
11		
12		

Total:	

Total Activity: _________ Min. Burned: ____________ Kcal

Water Intake

Week:____ From: To:

Weekly Summary

	MAEL	Activity	Calories Burned	Note
Sunday	😊 ☹️	😊 ☹️	😊 ☹️	
Monday	😊 ☹️	😊 ☹️	😊 ☹️	
Tuesday	😊 ☹️	😊 ☹️	😊 ☹️	
Wednesday	😊 ☹️	😊 ☹️	😊 ☹️	
Thursday	😊 ☹️	😊 ☹️	😊 ☹️	
Friday	😊 ☹️	😊 ☹️	😊 ☹️	
Saturday	😊 ☹️	😊 ☹️	😊 ☹️	

Note

www.ingramcontent.com/pod-product-compliance
Lightning Source LLC
Chambersburg PA
CBHW051816250726
48659CB00005B/1522